The Ultimate

Air Fryer Cookbook

Quick, Easy and Delicious Frying
Recipes for Quick and Easy Meals

Elma Boren

TABLE OF CONTENTS

INTRODUCTION

Air fryers are new appliance that have been gaining popularity in the last few years. Especially now with the holiday season approaching, many people are considering gifting an air fryer to someone they know who might not be aware of them.

Air fryers are great for frying food in a healthier way. Less oil is needed, and the food can be cooked without trans fats or other preservatives that are found in deep-fryers. However, air fryers also use hot air to cook more quickly. This means they should be used with caution by children and pets who may reach into them.

An air fryer is a cooking gadgets that has a wide variety of purposes; it can make french fries, roast beef or pumpkin pie crusts as well as pizza dough. Air frying takes only minutes to cook pieces of meat on the outer layer while keeping them juicy on the inside. The way air fryers work is by circulating hot air to cook the food.

The Cuisinart Air Fryer is a popular choice for an air fryer and can be bought through online shops or retail stores. The

Cuisinart Air Fryer can be bought as a standalone unit, or it can easily be attached to other Cuisinart products like the blender or food processor. The Air Fryer comes with a cookbook and has recipe cards available. It takes 19 minutes to prepare the air fryer and takes another 15 minutes for the food to cook.

The air fryer uses 0.2 gallons, or about 3 cups of oil, which is quite a bit more than regular deep-fryers do but still far less than the amount that would be needed if using a regular frying pan. This can be a problem if you need to keep on hand great amounts of cooking oils; however, it can save a lot of time since it takes only a few minutes to make french fries instead of frying them in small batches at different times.

BREAKFAST

1. Grilled Gruyere Cheese Sandwich

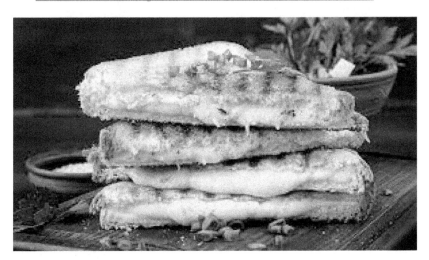

Preparation Time: 5 Minutes

Cooking Time: 10 Minutes

Servings: 1

Ingredients:

- 2 ounces of thinly sliced Gruyere cheese

- 2 slices of whole-grain bread

- 1 tablespoon of butter

Directions:

1. Lay the Gruyere cheese between the 2 slices of bread.

2. Butter up the outside of the bread slices.

3. Place the cheese sandwich in the air fryer basket. You may need to use toothpicks to secure.

4. Air fry the sandwich for approximately 3-5 minutes at 360 degrees F until the cheese melts.

5. Flip the sandwich over and turn the heat up to 380 degrees F until crisp.

6. Continue to air fryer for approximately 5 minutes, until the sandwich is to your desired texture. You will need to check continually that the sandwich doesn't burn.

7. Set to one side to cool slightly before enjoying.

Nutrition: Calories: 151 kcal Fat: 7.1g Carbs: 17.9g Protein: 3.6g

2. Pancakes

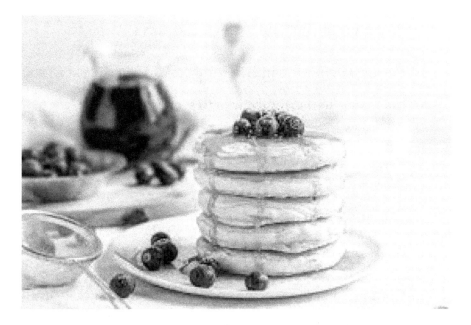

Preparation Time: 5 minutes

Cooking Time: 10 minutes

Servings: 2

Ingredients:

- 2 tbsps. coconut oil

- 1 tsp. maple extract

- 2 tbsps. cashew milk

- 2 eggs

- 2/3 oz. /20g pork rinds

Directions:

1. Grind up the pork rinds until fine and mix with the rest of the ingredients, except the oil.

2. Add the oil to a skillet. Add a quarter-cup of the batter and fry until golden on each side. Continue adding the remaining batter.

Nutrition: Calories: 280 Carbs: 31 g Fat: 2 g Protein: 5 g

3. Breakfast Sandwich

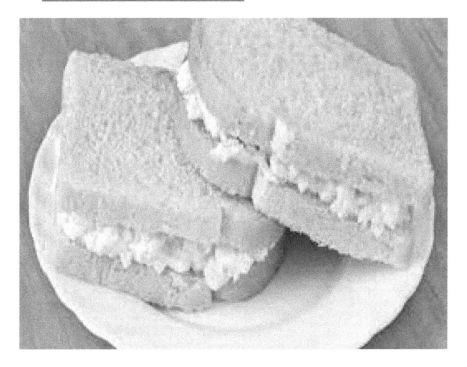

Preparation Time: 5 minutes

Cooking Time: 5 minutes

Servings: 1

Ingredients:

- 2 oz. /60g cheddar cheese

- 1/6 oz. /30g smoked ham

- 2 tbsps. butter

- 4 eggs

Directions:

1. Fry all the eggs and sprinkle the pepper and salt on them.

2. Place an egg down as the sandwich base. Top with the ham and cheese and a drop or two of Tabasco.

3. Place the other egg on top and enjoy.

Nutrition: Calories: 180 Carbs: 19 g Fat: 7 g Protein: 10 g

4. Air fryer Egg Muffins

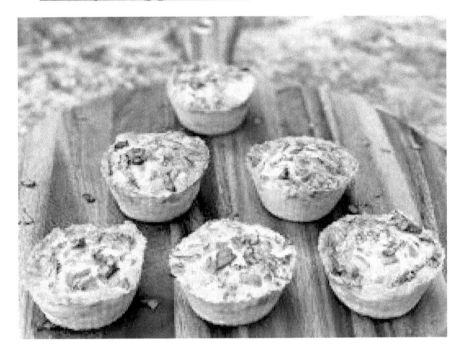

Preparation Time: 10 minutes

Cooking Time: 15-20 minutes

Servings: 1

Ingredients:

- 1 tbsp. green pesto

- Oz/75g shredded cheese

- Oz/150g cooked bacon

- 1 scallion, chopped

- Eggs

Directions:

1. You should set your fryer to 350°F/175°C.

2. Place liners in a regular cupcake tin. This will help with easy removal and storage.

3. Beat the eggs with pepper, salt, and the pesto. Mix in the cheese.

4. Pour the eggs into the cupcake tin and top with the bacon and scallion.

5. Cook for 15-20 minutes, or until the egg is set.

Nutrition: Calories: 160 Carbs: 11 g Fat: 6 g Protein: 8 g

5. Bacon & Eggs

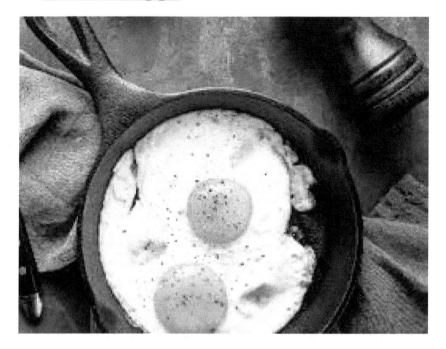

Preparation Time: 5 minutes

Cooking Time: 5 minutes

Servings: 1

Ingredients:

- Parsley

- Cherry tomatoes

- 1/3 oz. /150g bacon

- Eggs

Directions:

1. Fry up the bacon and put it to the side.

2. Scramble the eggs in the bacon grease, with some pepper and salt. If you want, scramble in some cherry tomatoes. Sprinkle with some parsley and enjoy.

Nutrition: Calories: 150 Carbs: 10 g Fat: 6 g Protein: 7 g

6. <u>Eggs on the Go</u>

Preparation Time: 5 minutes

Cooking Time: 15 minutes

Servings: 1

Ingredients:

- 110g bacon, cooked

- Pepper

- Salt

- Eggs

Directions:

1. You should set your fryer to 400°F/200°C.

2. Place liners in a regular cupcake tin. This will help with easy removal and storage.

3. Crack an egg into each of the cups and sprinkle some bacon onto each of them. Season with some pepper and salt.

4. Bake for 15 minutes, or once the eggs are set.

Nutrition: Calories: 140 Carbs: 10 g Fat: 5 g Protein: 7 g

7. Cream Cheese Pancakes

Preparation Time: 10 minutes

Cooking Time: 10 minutes

Servings: 1

Ingredients:

- 2 oz. cream cheese

- 2 eggs

- ½ tsp. cinnamon

- 1 tbsp coconut flour

- ½ to 1 packet of Sugar

Directions:

1. Mix together all the ingredients until smooth.

2. Heat up a non-stick skillet with butter or coconut oil on medium-high.

3. Make them as you would normally pancakes.

4. Cook it on one side and then flip to cook the other side!

5. Top with some butter and/or sugar.

Nutrition: Calories: 190 Carbs: 15 g Fat: 8 g Protein: 9 g

8. Breakfast Mix

Preparation Time: 5 minutes

Cooking Time: 10 minutes

Servings: 1

Ingredients:

- Tbsp coconut flakes, unsweetened

- Tbsp hemp seeds

- Tbsp flaxseed, ground

- 2 tbsp sesame, ground

- 2 tbsp cocoa, dark, unsweetened

Directions:

1. Grind the flaxseed with the sesame.

2. Make sure you grind the sesame seeds for a short time only.

3. Mix all of the ingredients in a jar and shake it to mix it well.

4. Keep refrigerated until ready to eat.

5. Serve softened with black coffee or even with still water and add coconut oil if you want to increase the fat content. It also blends well with mascarpone cheese or cream.

Nutrition: Calories: 175 Carbs: 13 g Fat: 6 g Protein: 8 g

9. Breakfast Muffins

Preparation Time: 10 minutes

Cooking Time: 15-20 minutes

Servings: 1

Ingredients:

- 1 medium egg

- ¼ cup heavy cream

- 1 slice cooked bacon (cured, pan-fried, cooked)

- 1 oz. cheddar cheese

- Salt and black pepper (to taste)

Directions:

1. Preheat your fryer to 350°F/175°C.

2. In a bowl, combine the eggs with the cream, salt and pepper.

3. Spread into muffin tins and fill the cups half full.

4. Place 1 slice of bacon into each muffin hole and half ounce of cheese on top of each muffin.

5. Bake for around 15-20 minutes or until slightly browned.

6. Add another ½ oz. of cheese onto each muffin and broil until the cheese is slightly browned. Serve!

Nutrition: Calories: 250 Carbs: 15 g Fat: 10 g Protein: 12 g

10. Egg Porridge

Preparation Time: 5 minutes

Cooking Time: 10 minutes

Servings: 1

Ingredients:

- 2 organic free-range eggs

- 1/3 cup organic heavy cream without food additives

- 2 packages of your preferred sweetener

- 2 tbsp grass-fed butter ground organic cinnamon to taste

Directions:

1. In a bowl add the eggs, cream and sweetener, and mix together.

2. Melt the butter in a saucepan over a medium heat. Lower the heat once the butter is melted.

3. Combine together with the egg and cream mixture.

4. While cooking, mix until it thickens and curdles.

5. When you see the first signs of curdling, remove the saucepan immediately from the heat.

6. Pour the porridge into a bowl. Sprinkle cinnamon on top and serve immediately.

Nutrition: Calories: 120 Carbs: 7 g Fat: 5 g Protein: 6 g

VEGETABLES AND SIDES

11. Eggplant stacks

Preparation Time: 5 minutes

Cooking Time: 15 minutes

Servings: 4

Ingredients:

- 2large tomatoes; cut into ¼-inch slices

- ¼ cup fresh basil, sliced

- 4oz. Fresh mozzarella; cut into ½-oz. Slices

- 1 medium eggplant; cut into ¼-inch slices

- 2tbsp. Olive oil

Directions:

1. In a 6-inch round baking dish, place four slices of eggplant on the bottom. Put a slice of tomato on each eggplant round, then mozzarella, then eggplant. Repeat as necessary.

2. Drizzle with olive oil. Cover dish with foil and place dish into the air fryer basket. Adjust the temperature to 350 degrees f and set the timer for 12 minutes.

3. When done, eggplant will be tender. Garnish with fresh basil to serve.

Nutrition: Calories: 195; Protein: 8.5g; Fiber: 5.2g; Fat: 12.7g; Carbs: 12.7g

12. Air Fried Spaghetti Squash

Preparation Time: 5 minutes

Cooking Time: 50 minutes

Servings: 4

Ingredients:

- ½ large spaghetti squash

- 2tbsp. Salted butter; melted.

- 1 tbsp. Coconut oil

- 1tsp. Dried parsley.

- ½tsp. Garlic powder.

Directions:

1. Brush shell of spaghetti squash with coconut oil. Place the skin side down and brush the inside with butter. Sprinkle with garlic powder and parsley.

2. Place squash with the skin side down into the air fryer basket. Adjust the temperature to 350 degrees f and set the timer for 30 minutes

3. When the timer beeps, flip the squash so skin side is up and cook an additional 15 minutes or until fork tender. Serve warm.

Nutrition: Calories: 182; Protein: 1.9g; Fiber: 3.9g; Fat: 11.7g; Carbs: 18.2g

13. Beets and Blue Cheese Salad

Preparation Time: 10 minutes

Cooking Time: 15 minutes

Servings: 6

Ingredients:

- 6beets, peeled and quartered

- Salt and black pepper to the taste

- ¼ cup blue cheese, crumbled

- 1 tablespoon olive oil

Directions:

1. Put beets in your air fryer, cook them at 350 degrees F for 14 minutes and transfer them to a bowl. Add blue cheese, salt, pepper and oil, toss and serve. Enjoy!

Nutrition: Calories 100, Fat 4, Fiber 4, Carbs 10, Protein 5

14. Broccoli Salad

Preparation Time: 10 minutes

Cooking Time: 10 minutes

Servings: 4

Ingredients:

- 1 broccoli head, with separated florets

- 1 tbsp. peanut oil

- 6cloves of garlic, minced

- 1 tbsp. Chinese rice wine vinegar

- Salt and black pepper to taste

Directions:

1. In a bowl, mix broccoli half of the oil with salt, pepper and, toss, transfer to your air fryer and cook at 350 degrees F for 8 minutes. Halfway through, shake the fryer. Take the broccoli out and put it into a salad bowl, add the rest of the peanut oil, garlic and rice vinegar, mix really well and serve. Enjoy!

Nutrition: Calories 121, Fat 3, Fiber 4, Carbs 4, Protein 4

15. Roasted Brussels Sprouts with Tomatoes

Preparation Time: 5 minutes

Cooking Time: 10 minutes

Servings: 4

Ingredients:

- 1-pound Brussels sprouts, trimmed

- Salt and black pepper to the taste

- 6cherry tomatoes, halved

- ¼ cup green onions, chopped

- 1 tablespoon olive oil

Directions:

1. Season Brussels sprouts with salt and pepper, put them in your air fryer and cook at 350 degrees F for 10 minutes. Transfer them to a bowl, add salt, pepper, cherry tomatoes, green onions and olive oil, toss well and serve. Enjoy!

Nutrition: Calories 121, Fat 4, Fiber 4, Carbs 11, Protein 4

16. Cheesy Brussels Sprouts

Preparation Time: 10 minutes

Cooking Time: 10 minutes

Servings: 4

Ingredients:

- 1-pound Brussels sprouts, washed

- Juice of 1 lemon

- Salt and black pepper to the taste

- 2tablespoons butter

- 3tablespoons parmesan, grated

Directions:

1. Put Brussels sprouts in your air fryer, cook them at 350 degrees F for 8 minutes and transfer them to a bowl. Warm up a pan over moderate heat with the butter, then add lemon juice, salt and pepper, whisk well and add to Brussels sprouts. Add parmesan, toss until parmesan melts and serve. Enjoy!

Nutrition: Calories 152, Fat 6, Fiber 6, Carbs 8, Protein 12

17. Sweet Baby Carrots Dish

Preparation Time: 10 minutes

Cooking Time: 10 minutes

Servings: 4

Ingredients:

- 2cups baby carrots

- A pinch of salt and black pepper

- 1 tablespoon brown sugar

- ½ tablespoon butter, melted

Directions:

1. In a dish that fits your air fryer, mix baby carrots with butter, salt, pepper and sugar, toss, introduce in your air fryer and cook at 350 degrees F for 10 minutes. Divide among plates and serve. Enjoy!

Nutrition: Calories 100, Fat 2, Fiber 3, Carbs 7, Protein 4

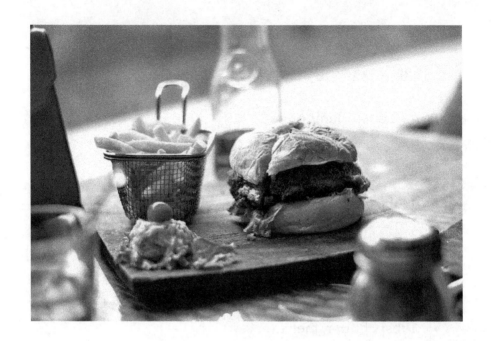

18. <u>Seasoned Leeks</u>

Preparation Time: 10 minutes

Cooking Time: 10 minutes

Servings: 4

Ingredients:

- 4leeks, washed, halved

- Salt and black pepper to taste

- 1 tbsp. butter, melted

- 1 tbsp. lemon juice

Directions:

1. Rub leeks with melted butter, season with salt and pepper, put in your air fryer and cook at 350 degrees F for 7 minutes. Arrange on a platter, drizzle lemon juice all over and serve. Enjoy!

Nutrition: Calories 100, Fat 4, Fiber 2, Carbs 6, Protein 2

19. Crispy Potatoes and Parsley

Preparation Time: 10 minutes

Cooking Time: 10 minutes

Servings: 4

Ingredients:

- 1-pound gold potatoes, cut into wedges

- Salt and black pepper to the taste

- 2tablespoons olive

- Juice from ½ lemon

- ¼ cup parsley leaves, chopped

Directions:

1. Rub potatoes with salt, pepper, lemon juice and olive oil, put them in your air fryer and cook at 350 degrees F for 10 minutes. Divide among plates, sprinkle parsley on top and serve. Enjoy!

Nutrition: Calories 152, Fat 3, Fiber 7, Carbs 17, Protein 4

20. Garlic Tomatoes

Preparation Time: 10 minutes

Cooking Time: 15 minutes

Servings: 4

Ingredients:

- 4garlic cloves, crushed
- 1-pound mixed cherry tomatoes
- 3thyme springs, chopped
- Salt and black pepper to the taste
- ¼ cup olive oil

Directions:

1. In a bowl, mix tomatoes with salt, black pepper, garlic, olive oil and thyme, toss to coat, introduce in your air fryer and cook at 360 degrees F for 15 minutes. Divide tomatoes mix on plates and serve. Enjoy!

Nutrition: Calories 100, Fat 0, Fiber 1, Carbs 1, Protein 6

MEAT

21. Sriracha Chicken Wings

Preparation Time: 10 minutes

Cooking Time: 35 minutes

Servings: 2

Ingredients:

- 1 lb. chicken wings

- 1/2 lime juice

- 1 tbsp grass-fed butter

- tbsp sriracha sauce

- 1/4 cup honey

Directions:

1 Preheat the air fryer to 182 C/ 360 F.

2 Add chicken wings in air fryer basket and cook for 30 minutes.

3 Meanwhile, in a pan, add all remaining ingredients and bring to boil for 3 minutes.

4   Once chicken wings are done then toss with sauce and
     serve.

Nutrition: Calories 711; Fat 32.6 g; Carbohydrates 35.9 g;
Sugar 35.8 g; Protein 65.8 g; Cholesterol 227 mg

22. Sweet & Spicy Chicken Wings

Preparation Time: 10 minutes

Cooking Time: 20 minutes

Servings: 8

Ingredients:

- lbs. chicken wings
- tbsp honey
- 1/2 cup buffalo sauce
- tbsp grass-fed butter, melted
- Salt and Pepper

Directions:

1   Put the chicken wings into the basket of the air fryer and cook for 20 minutes at 400 F/ 204 C. Shake air fryer basket 2 times during the cooking.

2   In a large bowl, combine together honey, buffalo sauce, butter, pepper, and salt.

3   Add cooked chicken wings into the bowl and toss until well coated with sauce.

4   Serve and enjoy.

Nutrition: Calories 262; Fat 11.7 g; Carbohydrates 4.6 g;Sugar 4.4 g; Protein 32.9 g; Cholesterol 109 mg

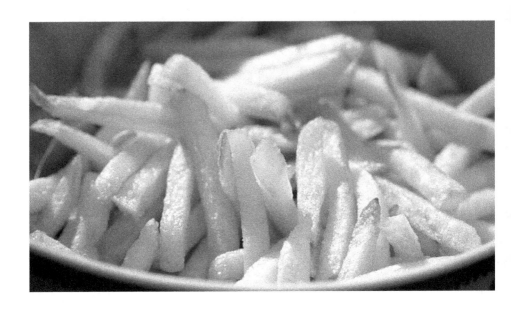

23. Ginger Garlic Chicken

Preparation Time: 10 minutes

Cooking Time: 30 minutes

Servings: 2

Ingredients:

- chicken thighs, skinless and boneless
- 1/2 tsp ground ginger
- 1 garlic clove, minced
- tbsp ketchup
- 1/2 cup honey

Directions:

1   Cut chicken thighs into the small pieces and place them into the air fryer basket and cook for 25 minutes at 390 F/ 198 C.

2   Meanwhile, in a pan heat together honey, ketchup, garlic, and ground ginger for 4-5 minutes.

3   Once the chicken is cooked then transfer into the mixing bowl.

4   Pour honey mixture over the chicken and toss until well coated.

5   Serve and enjoy.

Nutrition: Calories 554; Fat 16.3 g; Carbohydrates 37.2 g; Sugar 36.5 g; Protein 63.7 g; Cholesterol 195 mg

24. Salt and Pepper Wings

Preparation Time: 5 minutes

Cooking Time: 10 minutes

Servings: 4

Ingredients:

- 2 teaspoons salt

- 2 teaspoons fresh ground pepper

- 2 pounds chicken wings

Directions:

1. In a bowl, mix the salt and pepper.

2. Add the wings to the bowl and mix with your hands to coat every last one.

3. Put 8 to 10 wings in the air fryer basket that has been sprayed with nonstick cooking spray. Set for 350 degrees F (there is no need to preheat) and cook about 15 minutes, turning once at 7 minutes.

4. Repeat with rest of wings and serve hot.

Nutrition: Calories 342 Fat 14.8 g Carbohydrates 1 g Sugar 0 g

Protein 49.2 g Cholesterol 146 mg

25. Parmesan Chicken Wings

Preparation Time: 10 minutes

Cooking Time: 25 minutes

Serve: 4

Ingredients:

- 1 1/2 lbs. chicken wings
- 3/4 tbsp garlic powder
- 1/4 cup parmesan cheese, grated
- 2 tbsp arrowroot powder
- Salt and Pepper

Directions:

1. Preheat the air fryer to 380 F.

2. In a bowl, mix the garlic powder, parmesan cheese, arrowroot powder, pepper, and salt together. Add chicken wings and toss until well coated.

3. Put the chicken wings into the air fryer basket. Spray top of chicken wings with cooking spray.

4. Select chicken and press start. Shake air fryer basket halfway through.

5. Serve and enjoy.

Nutrition: Calories 386 Fat 15.3 g Carbohydrates 5.6 g Sugar 0.4 g Protein 53.5 g Cholesterol 160 mg

26. Western Chicken Wings

Preparation Time: 10 minutes

Cooking Time: 15 minutes

Serve: 4

Ingredients:

- 2 lbs. chicken wings
- 1 tsp Herb de Provence
- 1 tsp paprika
- 1/2 cup parmesan cheese, grated
- Salt and Pepper

Directions:

1. Add cheese, paprika, herb de Provence, pepper, and salt into the large mixing bowl. Place the chicken wings into the bowl and toss well to coat.

2. Preheat the air fryer to 350 F.

3. Place the chicken wings into the air fryer basket. Spray top of chicken wings with cooking spray.

4. Cook chicken wings for 15 minutes. Turn chicken wings halfway through.

5. Serve and enjoy.

Nutrition: Calories 473 Fat 19.6 g Carbohydrates 0.8 g Sugar 0.1 g Protein 69.7 g Cholesterol 211 mg

27. Perfect Chicken Thighs Dinner

Preparation Time: 10 minutes

Cooking Time: 15 minutes

Serve: 4

Ingredients:

- 4 chicken thighs, bone-in & skinless
- 1/4 tsp ground ginger
- 2 tsp paprika
- 2 tsp garlic powder
- salt and pepper

Directions:

1. Preheat the air fryer to 400 F.

2. In a bowl, mix ginger, paprika, garlic powder, pepper, and salt together and rub all over chicken thighs.

3. Spray chicken thighs with cooking spray.

4. Place chicken thighs into the air fryer basket and cook for 10 minutes.

5. Turn chicken thighs and cook for 5 minutes more.

6. Serve and enjoy.

Nutrition: Calories 286 Fat 11 g Carbohydrates 1.8 g Sugar 0.5 g Protein 42.7 g Cholesterol 130 mg

28. Perfectly Spiced Chicken Tenders

Preparation Time: 10 minutes

Cooking Time: 13 minutes

Serve: 4

Ingredients:

- 6 chicken tenders
- 1 tsp onion powder
- 1 tsp garlic powder
- 1 tsp paprika
- 1 tsp kosher salt

Directions:

1. Preheat the air fryer to 380 F.

2. In a bowl, mix onion powder, garlic powder, paprika, and salt together and rub all over chicken tenders.

3. Spray chicken tenders with cooking spray.

4. Place chicken tenders into the air fryer basket and cook for 13 minutes.

5. Serve and enjoy.

Nutrition: Calories 423 Fat 16.4 g Carbohydrates 1.5 g Sugar 0.5 g Protein 63.7 g Cholesterol 195 mg

29. Flavorful Steak

Preparation Time: 10 minutes

Cooking Time: 18 minutes

Serve: 2

Ingredients:

- 2 steaks, rinsed and pat dry
- ½ tsp garlic powder
- 1 tsp olive oil
- Pepper
- Salt

Directions:

1. Brush steaks with olive oil and season with garlic powder, pepper, and salt.

2. Preheat the instant vortex air fryer oven to 400 F.

3. Place steaks on air fryer oven pan and air fry for 10-18 minutes. Turn halfway through.

4. Serve and enjoy.

Nutrition: Calories 361 Fat 10.9 g Carbohydrates 0.5 g Sugar 0.2 g Protein 61.6 g Cholesterol 153 mg

30. Easy Rosemary Lamb Chops

Preparation Time: 10 minutes

Cooking Time: 6 minutes

Serve: 4

Ingredients:

- 4 lamb chops
- 2 tbsp dried rosemary
- ¼ cup fresh lemon juice
- Pepper
- Salt

Directions:

1. In a small bowl, mix together lemon juice, rosemary, pepper, and salt.

2. Brush lemon juice rosemary mixture over lamb chops.

3. Place lamb chops on air fryer oven tray and air fry at 400 F for 3 minutes.

4. Turn lamb chops to the other side and cook for 3 minutes more.

5. Serve and enjoy.

Nutrition: Calories 267 Fat 21.7 g Carbohydrates 1.4 g Sugar 0.3 g Protein 16.9 g Cholesterol 0 mg

FISH AND SEAFOOD

31. Cheese and Ham Patties

Preparation Time: 10 minutes

Cooking Time: 10 minutes

Servings: 4

Ingredients:

- 1 puff pastry sheet

- 4 handfuls mozzarella cheese, grated

- 4 teaspoons mustard

- 8 ham slices, chopped

Directions:

1. Spread out puff pastry on a clean surface and cut it in 12 squares.

2. Divide cheese, ham, and mustard on half of them, top with the other halves, and seal the edges.

3. Place all the patties in your air fryer's basket and cook at 370 degrees F for 10 minutes.

4. Divide the patties between plates and serve.

Nutrition: Calories 212, Fat 12, Fiber 7, Carbs 14, Protein 8

32. Air-Fried Seafood

Preparation Time: 10 minutes

Cooking Time: 10 minutes

Servings: 4

Ingredients:

- 1 lb. fresh scallops, mussels, fish fillets, prawns, shrimp

- 2 eggs, lightly beaten

- Salt and black pepper

- 1 cup breadcrumbs mixed with the zest of 1 lemon

- Cooking spray

Directions:

1. Clean the seafood as needed.

2. Dip each piece into the egg; and season with salt and pepper.

3. Coat in the crumbs and spray with oil.

4. Arrange into the air fryer and cook for 6 minutes at 4000 F. turning once halfway through.

5. Serve and Enjoy!

Nutrition: Calories: 133 Protein: 17.4 grams Fat: 3.1 grams Carbohydrates: 8.2 grams

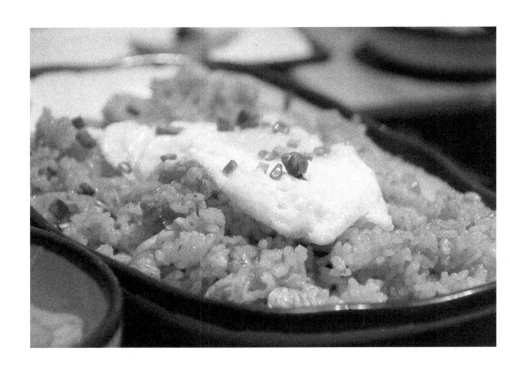

33. <u>Fish with Chips</u>

Preparation Time: 5 minutes

Cooking Time: 20 minutes

Servings: 2

Ingredients:

- 1 cod fillet (6 ounces)

- 3 cups salt

- 3 cups vinegar-flavored kettle cooked chips

- ¼ cup buttermilk

- salt and pepper to taste

Directions:

1. Mix to combine the buttermilk, pepper, and salt in a bowl. Put the cod and leave to soak for 5 minutes

2. Put the chips in a food processor and process until crushed. Transfer to a shallow bowl. Coat the fillet with the crushed chips.

3. Put the coated fillet in the air frying basket. Cook for 12 minutes at 4000 F.

4. Serve and Enjoy!

Nutrition: Calories: 646 Protein: 41 grams Fat: 33 grams Carbohydrates: 48 grams

34. Crumbly Fishcakes

Preparation Time: 5 minutes

Cooking Time: 10 minutes

Servings: 4

Ingredients:

- 8 oz. salmon, cooked

- 1 ½ oz. potatoes, mashed

- A handful of parsley, chopped

- Zest of 1 lemon

- 1 ¾ oz. plain flour

Directions:

1. Carefully flakes the salmon. In a bowl, mix flaked salmon, zest, capers, dill, and mashed potatoes.

2. From small cakes using the mixture and dust the cakes with flour; refrigerate for 60 minutes.

3. Preheat your air fryer to 3500 F. and cook the cakes for 7 minutes. Serve chilled.

Nutrition: Calories: 210 Protein: 10 grams Fat: 7 grams Carbohydrates: 25 grams

35. Bacon Wrapped with Shrimp

Preparation Time: 10 minutes

Cooking Time: 20 minutes

Servings: 4

Ingredients:

- 16 thin slices of bacon

- 16 pieces of tiger shrimp (peeled and deveined)

Directions:

1. With a slice of bacon, wrap each shrimp. Put all the finished pieces in tray and chill for 20 minutes.

2. Arrange the bacon-wrapped shrimp in the air frying basket. Cook for 7 minutes at 3900 F. Transfer to a plate lined with paper towels to drain before serving.

Nutrition: Calories: 436 Protein: 32 grams Fat: 41.01 grams Carbohydrates: 0.8 grams

36. Crab Legs

Preparation Time: 10 minutes

Cooking Time: 10 minutes

Servings: 4

Ingredients:

- 3 lb. crab legs

- ¼ cup salted butter, melted and divided

- ½ lemon, juiced

- ¼ tsp. garlic powder

Directions:

1. In a bowl, toss the crab legs and two tablespoons of the melted butter together. Place the crab legs in the basket of the fryer.

2. Cook at 400°F for fifteen minutes, giving the basket a good shake halfway through.

3. Combine the remaining butter with the lemon juice and garlic powder.

4. Crack open the cooked crab legs and remove the meat. Serve with the butter dip on the side, and enjoy!

Nutrition: Calories 272, Fat 19, Fiber 9, Carbs 18, Protein 12

37. Fish Sticks

Preparation Time: 5 minutes

Cooking Time: 10 minutes

Servings: 4

Ingredients:

- 1 lb. whitefish

- 2 tbsp. Dijon mustard

- ¼ cup mayonnaise

- 1 ½ cup pork rinds, finely ground

- ¾ tsp. Cajun seasoning

Directions:

1. Place the fish on a tissue to dry it off, then cut it up into slices about two inches thick.

2. In one bowl, combine the mustard and mayonnaise, and in another, the Cajun seasoning and pork rinds.

3. Coat the fish firstly in the mayo-mustard mixture, then in the Cajun-pork rind mixture. Give each slice a shake

to remove any surplus. Then place the fish sticks in the basket of the air flyer.

4. Cook at 400°F for five minutes. Turn the fish sticks over and cook for another five minutes on the other side.

5. Serve warm with a dipping sauce of your choosing and enjoy.

Nutrition: Calories 212, Fat 12, Fiber 7, Carbs 14, Protein 8

38. Crusty Pesto Salmon

Preparation Time: 5 minutes

Cooking Time: 10 minutes

Servings: 2

Ingredients:

- ¼ cup almonds, roughly chopped

- ¼ cup pesto

- 2 x 4-oz. salmon fillets

- 2 tbsp. unsalted butter, melted

Directions:

1. Mix the almonds and pesto together.

2. Place the salmon fillets in a round baking dish, roughly six inches in diameter.

3. Brush the fillets with butter, followed by the pesto mixture, ensuring to coat both the top and bottom. Put the baking dish inside the fryer.

4. Cook for twelve minutes at 390°F.

5. The salmon is ready when it flakes easily when prodded with a fork. Serve warm.

Nutrition: Calories 354 Fat 21 Carbs 23 Protein 19

39. Cajun Salmon

Preparation Time: 5 minutes

Cooking Time: 10 minutes

Servings: 4

Ingredients:

- 2 4-oz skinless salmon fillets

- 2 tbsp. unsalted butter, melted

- 1 pinch ground cayenne pepper

- 1 tsp. paprika

- ½ tsp. garlic pepper

Directions:

1. Using a brush, apply the butter to the salmon fillets.

2. Combine the other ingredients and massage this mixture into the fillets. Lay the fish inside your fryer.

3. Cook for seven minutes at 390°F.

4. When the salmon is ready it should flake apart easily.

5. Enjoy with the sides of your choosing.

Nutrition: Calories 383 Fat 12 Carbs 29 Protein 31

40. Buttery Cod

Preparation Time: 5 minutes

Cooking Time: 10 minutes

Servings: 4

Ingredients:

- 2 x 4-oz. cod fillets

- 2 tbsp. salted butter, melted

- 1 tsp. Old Bay seasoning

- ½ medium lemon, sliced

Directions:

1. Place the cod fillets in a dish.

2. Brush with melted butter, season with Old Bay, and top with some lemon slices.

3. Wrap the fish in aluminum foil and put into your fryer.

4. Cook for eight minutes at 350°F.

5. The cod is ready when it flakes easily. Serve hot.

Nutrition: Calories 354 Fat 21 Carbs 23 Protein 19

SNACKS AND DESSERT

41. Cherries and Rhubarb Bowls

Preparation Time: 10 minutes

Cooking Time: 35 minutes

Servings: 4

Ingredients:

- 2cups cherries, pitted and halved

- 1 cup rhubarb, sliced

- 1 cup apple juice

- 2tablespoons sugar

- ½ cup raisins.

Directions:

1. In a pot that fits your air fryer, combine the cherries with the rhubarb and the other ingredients, toss, cook at 330 degrees F for 35 minutes, divide into bowls, cool down and serve.

Nutrition: Calories – 212 Protein – 7 g Fat – 8 g Carbs – 13 g.

42. Pumpkin Bowls

Preparation Time: 10 minutes

Cooking Time: 15 minutes

Servings: 4

Ingredients:

- 2cups pumpkin flesh, cubed

- 1 cup heavy cream

- 1 teaspoon cinnamon powder

- 3tablespoons sugar

- 1 teaspoon nutmeg, ground

Directions:

1. In a pot that fits your air fryer, combine the pumpkin with the cream and the other ingredients, introduce in the fryer and cook at 360 degrees F for 15 minutes.

2. Divide into bowls and serve.

Nutrition: Calories – 212 Protein – 7 g Fat – 5 g Carbs – 15 g.

43. Apple Jam

Preparation Time: 10 minutes

Cooking Time: 25 minutes

Servings: 4

Ingredients:

- 1 cup water

- ½ cup sugar

- 1-pound apples, cored, peeled and chopped

- ½ teaspoon nutmeg, ground

Directions:

1. In a pot that suits your air fryer, mix the apples with the water and the other ingredients, toss, introduce the pan in the fryer and cook at 370 degrees F for 25 minutes.

2. Blend a bit using an immersion blender, divide into jars and serve.

Nutrition: Calories – 204 Protein – 4 g Fat – 3 g Carbs – 12 g.

44. Yogurt and Pumpkin Cream

Preparation Time: 10 minutes

Cooking Time: 30 minutes

Servings: 4

Ingredients:

- 1 cup yogurt

- 1 cup pumpkin puree

- 2eggs, whisked

- 2tablespoons sugar

- ½ teaspoon vanilla extract

Directions:

1. In a large bowl, mix the puree and the yogurt with the other ingredients, whisk well, pour into 4 ramekins, put them in the air fryer and cook at 370 degrees F for 30 minutes.

2. Cool down and serve.

Nutrition: Calories – 192 Protein – 4 g Fat – 7 g Carbs – 12 g.

45. Raisins Rice Mix

Preparation Time: 10 minutes

Cooking Time: 25 minutes

Servings: 6

Ingredients:

- 1 cup white rice

- 2cups coconut milk

- 3tablespoons sugar

- 1 teaspoon vanilla extract

- ½ cup raisins

Directions:

1. In the air fryer's pan, combine the rice with the milk and the other ingredients, introduce the pan in the fryer and cook at 320 degrees F for 25 minutes.

2. Divide into bowls and serve warm.

Nutrition: Calories – 132 Protein – 7 g Fat – 6 g Carbs – 11 g.

46. Orange Bowls

Preparation Time: 10 minutes

Cooking Time: 10 minutes

Servings: 4

Ingredients:

- 1 cup oranges, peeled and cut into segments

- 1 cup cherries, pitted and halved

- 1 cup mango, peeled and cubed

- 1 cup orange juice

- 2tablespoon sugar

Directions:

1. In the air fryer's pan, mix the oranges with the cherries and the other ingredients, toss and cook at 320 degrees F for 10 minutes.

2. Divide into bowls and serve cold.

Nutrition: Calories – 191 Protein – 4 g Fat – 7 g Carbs – 14 g.

47. Strawberry Jam

Preparation Time: 10 minutes

Cooking Time: 25 minutes

Servings: 8

Ingredients:

- 1 pound strawberries, chopped

- 1 tablespoon lemon zest, grated

- 1 and ½ cups water

- ½ cup sugar

- ½ tablespoon lemon juice

Directions:

1. In the air fryer's pan, mix the berries with the water and the other ingredients, stir, introduce the pan in your air fryer and cook at 330 degrees F for 25 minutes.

2. Divide into bowls and serve cold.

Nutrition: Calories – 202 Protein – 7 g Fat – 8 g Carbs – 6 g.

48. Caramel Cream

Preparation Time: 10 minutes

Cooking Time: 15 minutes

Servings: 4

Ingredients:

- 1 cup heavy cream
- 3tablespoons caramel syrup
- ½ cup coconut cream
- 1 tablespoon sugar
- ½ teaspoon cinnamon powder

Directions:

1. In a bowl, mix the cream with the caramel syrup and the other ingredients, whisk, divide into small ramekins, introduce in the fryer and cook at 320 degrees F and bake for 15 minutes.

2. Divide into bowls and serve cold.

Nutrition: Calories – 234 Protein – 5 g Fat – 13 g Carbs – 11 g.

49. Wrapped Pears

Preparation Time: 10 minutes

Cooking Time: 15 minutes

Servings: 4

Ingredients:

- 4puff pastry sheets
- 14ounces vanilla custard
- 2pears, halved
- 1 egg, whisked
- 2tbsp. sugar

Directions:

1. Put the puff pastry slices on a clean surface, add spoonful of vanilla custard in the center of each, top with pear halves and wrap.

2. Brush pears with egg, sprinkle sugar and place them in your air fryer's basket and cook at 320 °F for 15 minutes.

3. Divide parcels on plates and serve.

Nutrition: Calories – 200 Protein – 6 g Fat – 7 g Carbs – 6 g.

50. Perfect Cinnamon Toast

Preparation Time: 10 minutes

Cooking Time: 5 minutes

Servings: 6

Ingredients:

- 2 tsp. pepper

- 1 ½ tsp. cinnamon

- ½ C. sweetener of choice

- 1 C. coconut oil

- 12 slices whole wheat bread

Directions:

1. Melt coconut oil and mix with sweetener until dissolved. Mix in remaining ingredients minus bread till incorporated.

2. Spread mixture onto bread, covering all area.

3. Pour the coated pieces of bread into the Oven rack/basket. Place the Rack on the middle-shelf of the

Air fryer oven. Set temperature to 400°F, and set time to 5 minutes.

4. Remove and cut diagonally. Enjoy!

Nutrition: Calories – 124 Protein – 0 g Fat – 2 g Carbs – 5 g.

CONCLUSION

A ir fryers use hot air to replicate the traditional browning of foods Instead of submerging the food in oil. Similarly to searing, properly arranged foods are young, succulent, vibrantly dark-colored, and delectable.

An air-fryer cooker or appliance is a convection oven that is smaller than it appears – to be precise, a conservative round and hollow ledge convection oven (have a go at saying that multiple times quick

This is the healthiest way to cook food, and everyone in the family will love it and keep coming back for more without even realizing they are eating healthier.

You now have all of the information you need to get started with your air fryer! Simply choose a recipe to get started cooking with low sodium and low carbs in no time. Remember that eating safe doesn't mean you have to slave in the kitchen or spend a lot of money for hand-delivered meals. All you have to do is try fresh, tasty recipes that will quickly become family classics. Your air fryer will quickly become your most used kitchen appliance!

From now on, I believe you can rely on this book to help you solve those obstacles because you already know how to make the same thing healthier in the shortest amount of time. I'm not boasting about it at all. Many chefs agree that using an air fryer makes it healthier and faster. This isn't even an oven substitute; it's a one-of-a-kind experience in terms of cooking. We now have a large number of recipes to choose from, which I believe will enable us to expand our culinary horizons. It's also something you can depend on while you're on holiday. Since it thoroughly cooks the food, you can rely on it while relaxing in a recreational vehicle while listening to your favorite music. For all of these reasons, as well as a slew of others, I have faith in the air fryer and the flavor that the recipes can deliver.